Pooh's Little Fitness Book

**Look out for these rather less exhausting
Little titles from Methuen**

Available from all good bookshops

INSPIRED BY *A. A. Milne*

POOH'S LITTLE
FITNESS BOOK

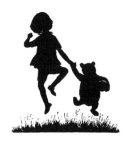

DECORATIONS BY *Ernest H. Shepard*

METHUEN

First published in Great Britain in 1997 by Methuen
an imprint of Reed International Books Limited
Michelin House, 81 Fulham Road, London SW3 6RB
and Auckland, Melbourne, Singapore and Toronto
Published in the United States 1996 by Dutton Children's Books
a division of Penguin Books USA, Inc.
Copyright © 1996 by the Trustees of the Pooh Properties
This presentation © 1996 by Dutton Children's Books
Text by A.A. Milne and illustrations by E.H. Shepard
from *When We Were Very Young, Winnie-the-Pooh, Now We Are Six,*
and *The House At Pooh Corner*
Copyright under the Berne Convention
Written by Melissa Dorfman France Designed by Adrian Leichter

Printed in China

ISBN 0 416 19419 2

1 3 5 7 9 10 8 6 4 2

Contents

Introduction

A bear, however hard he tries,
Grows tubby without exercise. . . .
He thought: "If only I were thin!
But how does anyone begin?"

Embarking on an exercise program is indeed a daunting task. But in these fitness-conscious times, most of us cannot help feeling that it is the Thing to Do.

Fortunately, those who cringe at the thought of working out can take comfort and inspiration from this Very Useful Book, in which Pooh and his friends illustrate how easily exercise can be incorporated into one's daily routine. Readers will be pleasantly surprised to discover the fitness benefits of such ordinary activities as Balloon Gliding (which strengthens the upper body), Fir-cone Gathering (a tummy tightener), and Bouncing (an excellent aerobic exercise).

Filled with exercises and workout tips from the residents of the Hundred Acre Wood, this book contains all the Do's and Don't's of fitness in the Forest, and will teach the Astute Reader what many already know: that the best exercise is a lot like Pooh—short, slow, and always with a snack in sight.

Stretching and Warming Up

He had made up a little hum that very morning . . . in front of the glass: Tra-la-la, tra-la-la, *as he stretched up as high as he could go.*

—*Winnie-the-Pooh*

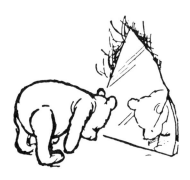

It is important to warm up before exercising. Stretching is an easy way to do so. (If you have no intention of exercising, a good stretch is also a nice way to warm up for a nap or a little mouthful of something.)

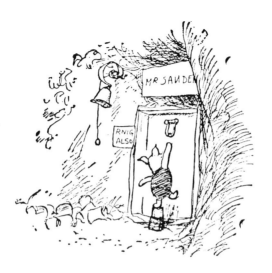

<u>DO</u> turn your simplest activities into opportunities for stretching. For instance, when visiting the home of a friend who is taller than you, stretch while reaching for the door knocker. Make sure to repeat with the other arm.

<u>DON'T</u> stretch too vigorously. Gentle, gradual stretching is best.

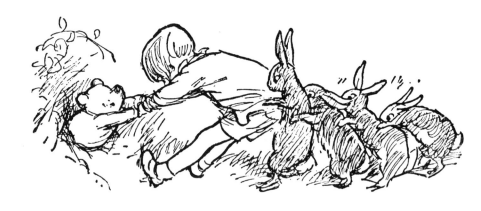

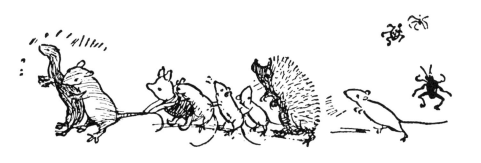

POOH'S STRETCHING TIP:
Stretching for a jar of honey
on the top shelf of the larder is an
enjoyable exercise—especially
around elevenish.

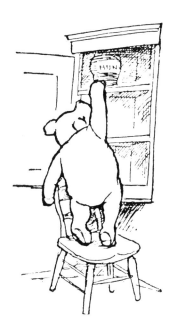

Cross-Training

At first Pooh and Rabbit and Piglet walked together, and Tigger ran round them in circles, and then, when the path got narrower, Rabbit, Piglet and Pooh walked one after another, and Tigger ran round them in oblongs, and by-and-by . . . Tigger ran up and down in front of them, and sometimes he bounced into Rabbit.

—*The House At Pooh Corner*

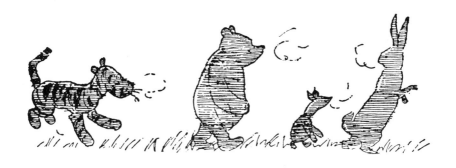

Cross-training, that popular and effective method of getting fit by doing different kinds of exercise on different days, is perfectly suited to life in the Hundred Acre Wood. Do a variety of the following activities vigorously and regularly, and you will be on your way to physical fitness. Walk to a friend's house, search for the North Pole, climb a tree . . .

⑤ WALKING ⑤

In any place and in any season, walking is a fine full-body workout. Walk briskly and breathe deeply to maximize the benefit to your heart, lungs, and muscles. Having a specific destination, such as Owl's house for a Proper Tea, is helpful. A lively Hum can help you keep up the pace.

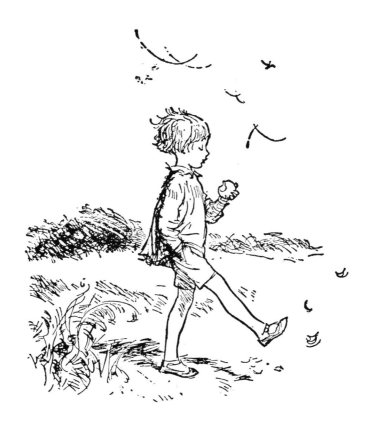

19

<u>DO</u> walk with a friend on a regular basis. That way, you are more likely to stick to your exercise regimen. Besides, it's so much more friendly with two.

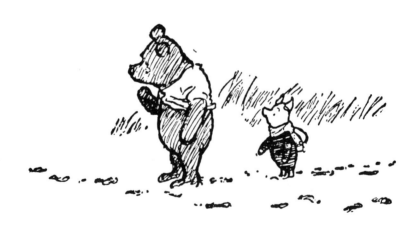

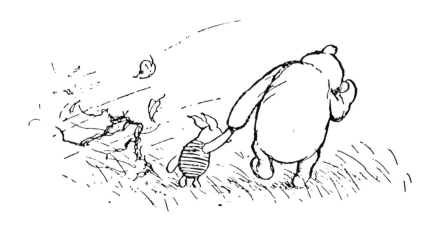

<u>DON'T</u> cancel a walk because of bad weather. If prepared with proper outdoor attire, you will rarely find the Atmospheric Conditions unfavorable to walking. In fact, walking against the wind provides a particularly beneficial workout.

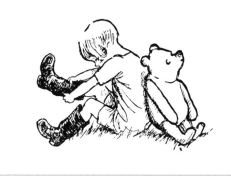

CHRISTOPHER ROBIN'S WALKING TIP:
To make a walk especially
exciting, pull on your Big Boots, invite
everybody, and call it an Expedition.
(Don't forget to bring Provisions.)

ഗ TREE CLIMBING ഗ

Excellent for strengthening and toning both the upper and lower body, this particular activity comes easily to some, but can be risky for others. Even the most experienced climbers risk a Very Bad Accident if a branch breaks.

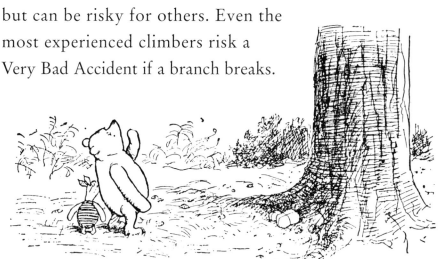

<u>DO</u> climb slowly and carefully, no matter how eager you are to reach the top of the tree (or the honey that may be there).

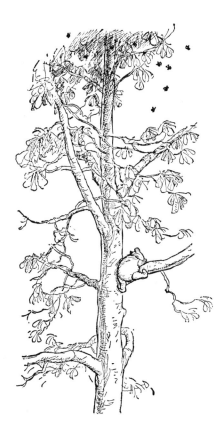

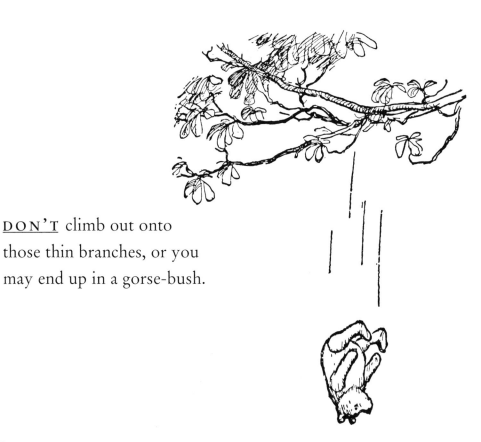

<u>**DON'T**</u> climb out onto
those thin branches, or you
may end up in a gorse-bush.

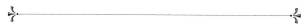

TIGGER'S TREE-CLIMBING TIP:
If you are a Tigger, keep in mind
that you can only climb upward, not downward,
or your tail will get in the way. Try to remember
this *before* reaching the top of a tree.

ཉ STRING CLIMBING ཉ

This is another excellent and exhilarating full-body work-out. It can also be a Very Useful Skill to have in an emergency—for instance, if your house blows down and you find that the door is now in the ceiling.

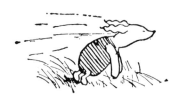

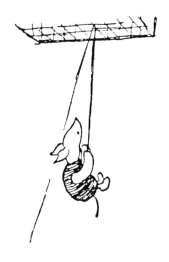

<u>DO</u> be sure to have at least two friends on the ground below, holding on to your string. Also, have extra string in case the first one breaks.

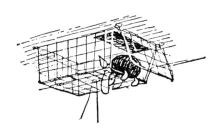

DON'T yell "Look at *me!*" at your support crew as you make your ascent. In the long run, you will be better off if they keep their eyes (and hands) on your string.

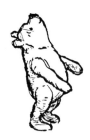

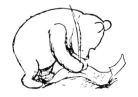

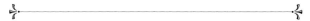

PIGLET'S STRING-CLIMBING TIP:
If you feel yourself beginning
to blinch, remember that your climb will be
a Very Grand Thing to talk about afterward.
Perhaps someone will even write a
Respectful Pooh Song about it.

SWIMMING & OTHER AQUATIC EXERCISES

Invigorating on a cool day and refreshing on a warm one, aquatic exercise is a delightful way to tone and strengthen muscles and can be enjoyed by anyone—which is not to say, however, that everyone will enjoy it.

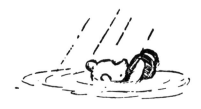

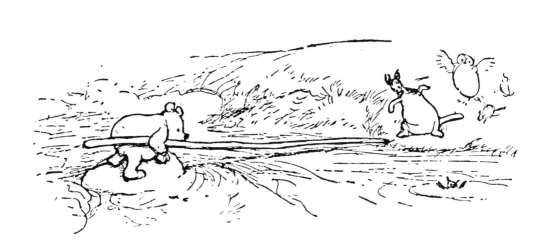

<u>DO</u> use the "more friendly with two" system when swimming. Keep an eye on your friend at all times so that you can lend a hand (or paw) should Sudden and Temporary Immersion occur.

<u>DON'T</u> swim for so long in a stream, river, or unheated pool that your tail becomes numb.

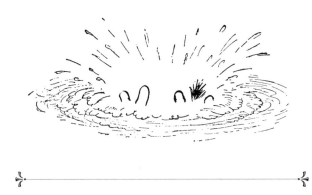

EEYORE'S SWIMMING TIP:
Learn to dive as well as swim.
Otherwise, you may not be able to avoid being
struck heavily on the chest by large stones
that somebody may drop on you.

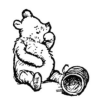

POOH'S AQUATIC-EXERCISE TIP:

A honey jar works well as a floating device.
Use your biggest jar, and cork it up tight. Of course, you
will want to empty the jar thoroughly first.

Aerobics

*Suddenly Winnie-the-Pooh stopped and pointed
excitedly in front of him. "Look!"*

*"What?" said Piglet, with a jump. And then, to
show that he hadn't been frightened, he jumped up
and down once or twice in an exercising
sort of way.*

—*Winnie-the-Pooh*

In addition to cross-training by walking, climbing, and swimming, you may seek a more intense workout. Several—though by no means all—of the residents of the Hundred Acre Wood do aerobic activities quite regularly.

ᔒ JUMPING ᔒ

One of the most widely practiced forms of exercise in the Forest, jumping is fun for both young and old and can be done almost anywhere. Jumping does not come as naturally to some (such as Kanga) as it does to others (such as Rabbit). But it is easily mastered with a little practice.

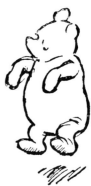

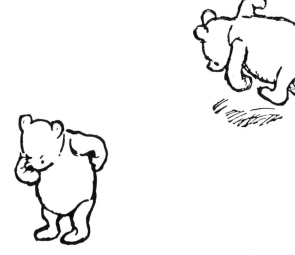

41

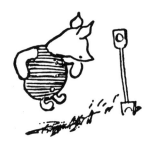

<u>DO</u> some vigorous jumping throughout the day whenever the opportunity arises. For instance, jump energetically on haycorns after planting them.

<u>DON'T</u> forget to watch where you are jumping, especially in the sandy part of the Forest, or you may fall down a mouse-hole.

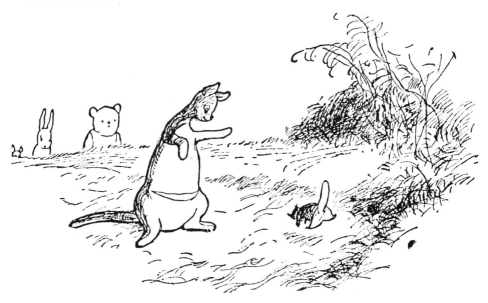

KANGA'S JUMPING TIP:

If you are too busy to set aside
a regular time for exercise, simply jump
instead of walk to wherever you're going.
For a more strenuous workout, put some
sort of weight in your pocket first.

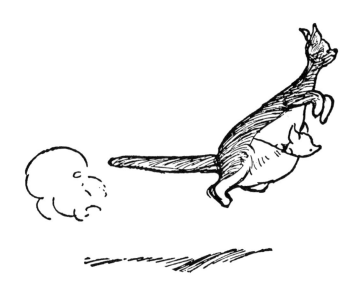

❦ BOUNCING ❦

Not to be confused with jumping, which is a more purposeful activity, bouncing is really an expression of exuberance and a natural state of being—for some. But it is also an excellent aerobic exercise.

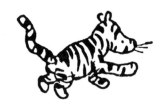

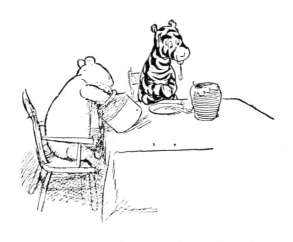

<u>DO</u> make sure to eat a healthful, well-balanced breakfast —preferably one low in fat and high in carbohydrates— before embarking on a vigorous day of calorie-burning bouncing.

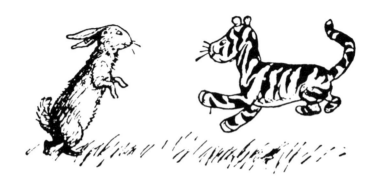

<u>DON'T</u> bounce so much in the company of others that they make plans to unbounce you by losing you in the Forest.

Avoid bouncing behind someone on the
slippery bank of a river, unless you are certain
that the someone wants a swim.

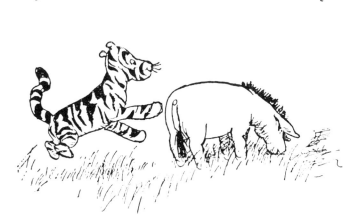

⑤ RUNNING ⑤

Running is among the most strenuous of aerobic activities. That is probably why it is practiced infrequently by Pooh and his friends. Nonetheless, running provides an excellent workout (and a good way of ensuring that one is not late for tea).

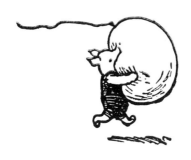

<u>DO</u> watch your step while running, or you may put your
foot in a rabbit hole.

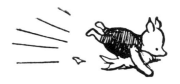

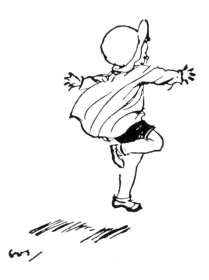

<u>DON'T</u> run so fast that you cannot enjoy the nice weather or the scenery around you. A trot, skip, or hoppity-hop is sufficient.

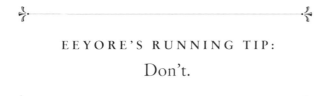

EEYORE'S RUNNING TIP:

Don't.

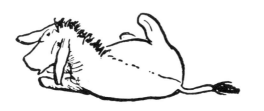

Workouts for Problem Areas

Owl explained about the Necessary Dorsal Muscles. He had explained this to Pooh and Christopher Robin once before, and had been waiting ever since for a chance to do it again, because it is a thing which you can easily explain twice before anybody knows what you are talking about.

—*The House At Pooh Corner*

Almost everyone wants to slim down, build up, or define a particular part of the body. Luckily, any number of the common and Useful activities briefly discussed here can also serve as exercises for arms, paws, wings, and/or tummies.

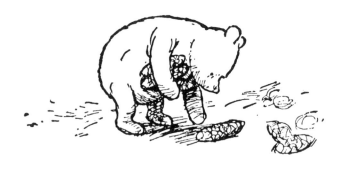

• **Fir-cone and Stick Gathering**—Trims the waist and tightens the tummy. Repeat at least a dozen times so that you will have enough cones and sticks for a game of Poohsticks afterward.

• **Digging**—A fine arm, chest, and shoulder exercise, during which you can also Accomplish Something, like making a Cunning Trap for Heffalumps.

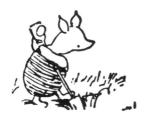

• **Balloon Gliding**—Not only strengthens the arms but may fill the stomach—if you glide near enough to a honey tree.

<u>DO</u> check the weather conditions before gliding. If there is insufficient wind, you will simply float up into the sky—and stay there.

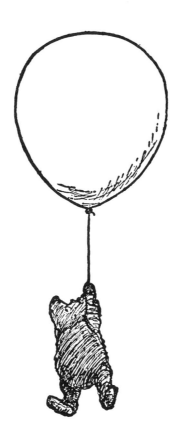

59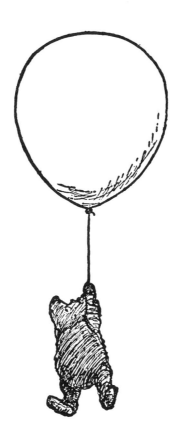

<u>DON'T</u> glide for too long a period of time on your first out-ing. Stiffness of the arms—for a week or longer—may result.

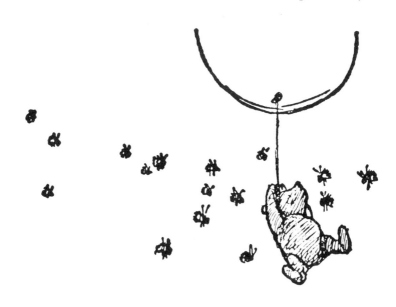

POOH'S BALLOON-GLIDING TIP:

If you roll around in a muddy place and
use a blue balloon, the bees may mistake you
for a small black cloud in a blue sky.
(Then again, they may not.)

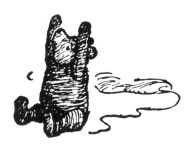

• **Flying**—Alternate strong flapping with periods of gliding in order to fully exercise the wings. But keep in mind that flying with a passenger, however Small an Animal, requires the Necessary Dorsal Muscles.

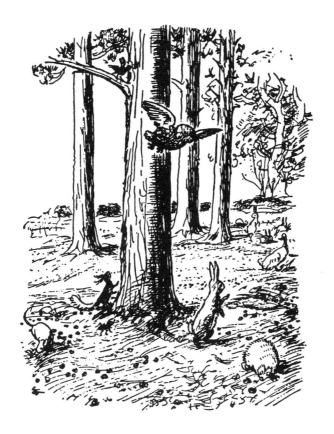

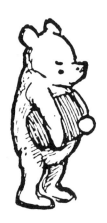

• **Honey-Jar Carrying and Lifting**—Carrying a full jar of honey provides a total-body workout. Lifting the jar above your shoulders is an effective way to tone your arms (or, of course, to lighten the jar).

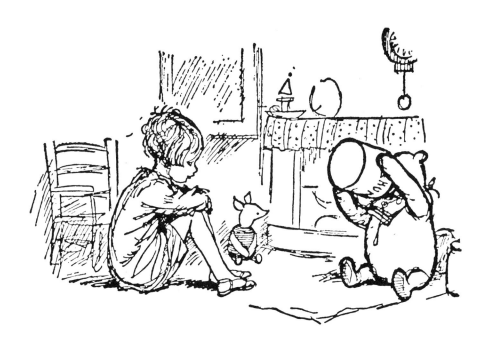

• **Stoutness Exercises**—Particularly popular with Pooh, who does them quite regularly—though unfortunately not as regularly as he does Honey-Jar Lifting.

<u>DO</u> reach up as high as you can before bending at the waist and reaching for the floor.

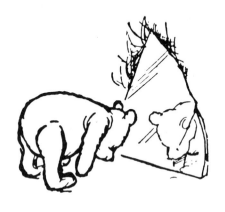

<u>DON'T</u> reach and bend too rapidly. Otherwise, you may find yourself saying, "Oh, help!" as you try to touch your toes.

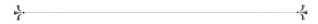

POOH'S STOUTNESS-EXERCISE TIP:
Sometimes, during exercise, a Hum
may come into your head. Wait for it patiently,
and remember that hums aren't things which
you get, they're things which get *you*.

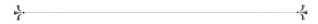

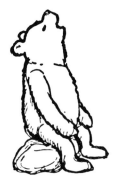

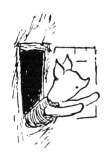

• **Bottle Throwing**—Good for toning and strengthening of arms or paws, but only really Useful when one is Surrounded by Water and in need of sending a Missage.

Cooling Down

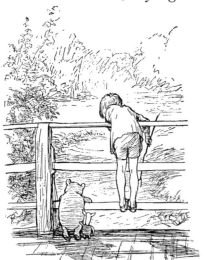

For a long time they looked at the river beneath them, saying nothing, and the river said nothing too, for it felt very quiet and peaceful on this summer afternoon.

—*The House At Pooh Corner*

Just as the body needs to warm up before a workout, it needs to cool down afterward. Like many residents of the Hundred Acre Wood, you may find that this is the most enjoyable part of your fitness regimen.

ꕥ TAIL TWITCHING ꕥ

This is a good way to slow the pace of your workout and begin to cool down. Twitch your tail left and then right, up and then down.

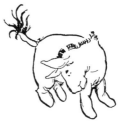

<u>DO</u> turn your head
and stretch your neck so
that you can see your tail as you
twitch it in each direction.

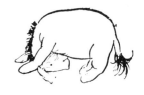

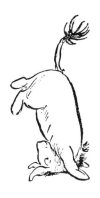

<u>DON'T</u> twitch too energetically, or you may find that you are frisking—which, while pleasant, isn't a good way to cool down.

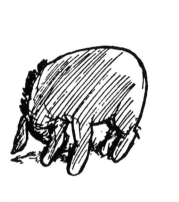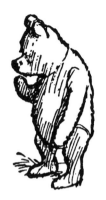

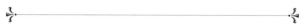

EEYORE'S TAIL-TWITCHING TIP:
Don't lose your tail, or you will have
nothing to twitch, unless someone can be
bothered to find it for you.

ଵ DANDELION BLOWING ଵ

While holding a dandelion, inhale slowly and deeply, then exhale slowly but forcefully, trying to blow away as many of the dandelion's seeds as possible. (This is also a Useful way to find out whether something will happen this year, next year, sometime, or never.)

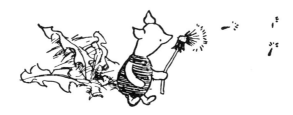

⑨ DEEP BREATHING ⑨

Find a comfortable spot to sit, close your eyes, and breathe slowly and deeply. Listening to the sounds of the Forest or singing a little Hum while you cool down encourages total muscle relaxation.

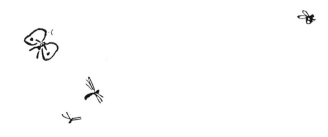

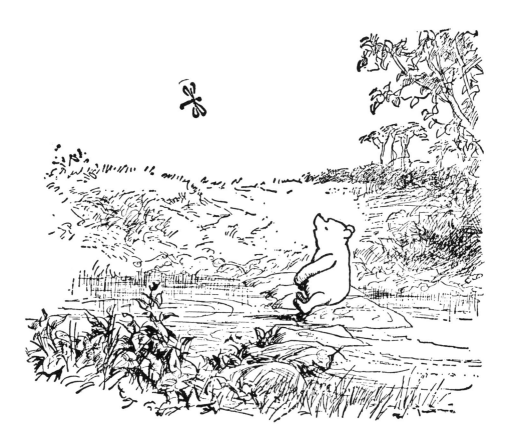

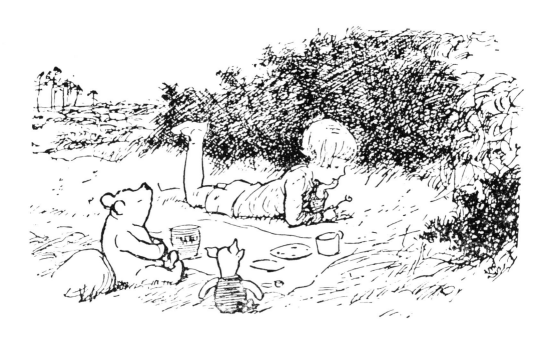

POOH'S POST-WORKOUT TIP:
The best way to revive yourself
after exercise—or any other activity—
is by having a little smackerel of
something with your friends.

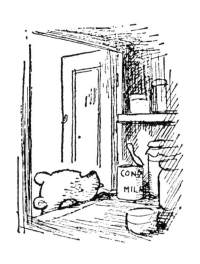